Therapeutic Fasting

Unlocking the Healing Powers of Abstinence

PROMISE ADEBAYO

This Book is dedicated to all those who embark on the profound journey of self-discovery and well-being through therapeutic fasting.

To the seekers of optimal health, may this guide illuminate your path and provide insights that empower your choices.

To the advocates of mindful living, may the principles within these pages resonate, fostering a deeper connection with your body and a harmonious relationship with the transformative practice of therapeutic fasting.

To the trailblazers of well-being, may this dedication stand as a tribute to your commitment to health, resilience, and the continuous pursuit of a balanced and vibrant life.

May your fasting journey be a source of inspiration, growth, and well-being, and may the knowledge within these pages be a guiding light on your transformative path.

With gratitude and well wishes,

PROMISE ADEBAYO

TABLE OF CONTENTS

INTRODUCTION:

In the relentless pursuit of optimal well-being, individuals are increasingly turning to ancient practices that resonate with timeless wisdom. Among these, therapeutic fasting emerges as a compelling avenue for unlocking the profound healing powers inherent in the simple act of abstinence. This eBook, "Therapeutic Fasting: Unlocking the Healing Powers of Abstinence," serves as your comprehensive guide to understanding, embracing, and harnessing the transformative potential of therapeutic fasting.

1. A Brief Overview of the Concept of Therapeutic Fasting:

At its essence, therapeutic fasting transcends the mere notion of abstaining from food; it is a deliberate and strategic approach to temporarily refraining from caloric intake for the betterment of one's health. Rooted in the age-old practice of allowing the body to rest and rejuvenate, therapeutic fasting is a holistic journey towards achieving physical, mental, and emotional balance.

2. Historical Context and Cultural Significance:

Delving into the historical annals reveals that fasting is not a mere contemporary health trend; rather, it is a practice deeply ingrained in various cultures and religions throughout human history. From ancient civilizations to religious traditions, fasting has played a multifaceted role, ranging from spiritual purification to physical healing. This section will explore the rich tapestry of fasting's historical context, shedding light on its cultural significance and the enduring impact it has had on diverse societies.

3. The Growing Interest in Fasting for Health Benefits:

In our modern age, marked by an ever-accelerating pace of life, the resurgence of interest in therapeutic fasting is palpable. As scientific research continues to unveil the intricate mechanisms behind fasting's impact on the human body, a groundswell of individuals seeks to harness its potential for enhanced well-being. From weight management to cognitive clarity, the growing body of evidence supporting the myriad health benefits of fasting has fueled a renewed enthusiasm for this ancient practice.

Embark on this enlightening journey with me as we explore the art and science of therapeutic fasting, uncovering the secrets that lie within the deliberate pause of nourishment—a pause that has the potential to revitalize the body, mind, and spirit. Welcome to a realm where the act of abstaining becomes a gateway to unlocking the profound healing powers that reside within us all.

CHAPTER 1: UNDERSTANDING THERAPEUTIC FASTING

1. DEFINITION AND TYPES OF THERAPEUTIC FASTING:

1.1 Defining Therapeutic Fasting:

At its core, therapeutic fasting is a deliberate and controlled period of abstaining from caloric intake, designed to facilitate the body's natural healing processes. It goes beyond traditional notions of intermittent fasting, evolving into a strategic approach aimed at promoting overall health and well-being.

1.2 Types of Therapeutic Fasting:

Within the realm of therapeutic fasting, various approaches cater to individual preferences and health goals. Some common types include intermittent fasting, water fasting, juice fasting, and partial fasting. Each type carries its own set of guidelines, benefits, and considerations, providing individuals with a range of options to tailor their fasting experience to suit their unique needs.

2. DIFFERENT FASTING DURATIONS AND APPROACHES:

2.1 Intermittent Fasting:

This approach involves cycling between periods of eating and fasting. Common methods include the 16/8 method (16 hours of fasting, 8 hours of eating) or the 5:2 method (five days of regular eating, two days of restricted caloric intake). Understanding the principles behind intermittent fasting allows individuals to integrate it seamlessly into their lifestyles.

2.2 Extended Water Fasting:

For those seeking more prolonged benefits, extended water fasting involves consuming only water for an extended period, typically ranging from 24 hours to several days. This deep dive into fasting requires careful preparation, monitoring, and adherence to safety guidelines, as the body undergoes significant physiological changes during this process.

2.3 Juice Fasting:

Juice fasting involves the consumption of fresh fruit and vegetable juices while abstaining from solid food. This approach provides essential nutrients while still allowing the digestive system to rest. However, understanding the balance between nutritional intake and caloric restriction is crucial to maximize the benefits of juice fasting.

3. THE SCIENCE BEHIND FASTING AND ITS IMPACT ON THE BODY:

3.1 Metabolic Shifts:

Fasting induces a shift in the body's energy source, transitioning from glucose to stored fat. This metabolic switch triggers ketosis, a state where the body efficiently burns fat for fuel, leading to weight loss and enhanced fat metabolism.

3.2 Cellular Repair and Autophagy:

One of the profound effects of fasting is the activation of autophagy, a cellular recycling process. During this phase, the body breaks down and removes damaged cells, promoting cellular repair and regeneration.

3.3 Hormonal Balance:

Fasting influences hormonal levels, including insulin and growth hormone. Improved insulin sensitivity and increased growth hormone secretion contribute to enhanced fat burning, muscle preservation, and overall metabolic health.

3.4 Inflammatory Reduction:

Fasting has been linked to a reduction in inflammation markers. This anti-inflammatory effect may contribute to improved cardiovascular health and a lower risk of chronic diseases.

Understanding the diverse physiological responses to therapeutic fasting is essential for individuals embarking on this transformative journey. In the following chapters, we will explore the specific benefits of therapeutic fasting, equipping readers with the knowledge needed to make informed decisions about integrating this powerful practice into their lives.

CHAPTER 2: BENEFITS OF THERAPEUTIC FASTING

1. WEIGHT MANAGEMENT AND METABOLIC IMPROVEMENTS:

Therapeutic fasting emerges as a powerful tool for individuals seeking effective weight management and metabolic enhancements. By inducing a metabolic shift towards fat utilization, fasting promotes weight loss and helps break the cycle of unhealthy eating habits. The process of ketosis, triggered during fasting, not only aids in shedding excess pounds but also contributes to improved metabolic flexibility, leading to long-term benefits in maintaining a healthy weight.

2. CELLULAR REPAIR AND AUTOPHAGY:

A fascinating aspect of therapeutic fasting lies in its ability to initiate cellular repair and autophagy. As the body enters a fasting state, cellular mechanisms are activated to break down and recycle damaged components. This process promotes overall cellular rejuvenation, contributing to improved longevity, enhanced immune function, and a reduced risk of various age-related diseases. The cellular renewal unleashed by fasting becomes a cornerstone for achieving optimal health.

3. COGNITIVE BENEFITS AND

MENTAL CLARITY:

Beyond its impact on the physical body, therapeutic fasting holds promise for cognitive health. Fasting has been associated with increased production of brain-derived neurotrophic factor (BDNF), a protein crucial for cognitive function and the formation of new neurons. Many individuals report heightened mental clarity, improved focus, and a sense of increased alertness during fasting periods. These cognitive benefits underscore the interconnectedness of fasting's effects on both body and mind.

4. BALANCING BLOOD SUGAR LEVELS AND INSULIN SENSITIVITY:

Therapeutic fasting plays a pivotal role in regulating blood sugar levels and enhancing insulin sensitivity. By reducing the frequency of meals and periods of caloric intake, fasting helps prevent insulin resistance—a key factor in the development of type 2 diabetes. This balanced approach to blood sugar management not only supports overall metabolic health but also mitigates the risk of chronic diseases associated with insulin dysregulation.

5. DETOXIFICATION AND IMPROVED GUT HEALTH:

Fasting serves as a natural detoxification process, allowing the body to expel accumulated toxins and metabolic byproducts. The reduction in food intake provides the digestive system with a much-needed break, diverting energy towards cellular repair and toxin elimination. Moreover, fasting promotes the growth of beneficial gut bacteria, fostering a healthier microbiome. This symbiotic relationship between fasting and gut health contributes to improved digestion, nutrient absorption, and overall gastrointestinal well-being.

As we delve deeper into the benefits of therapeutic fasting, it becomes evident that its impact extends far beyond weight management. The intricate interplay of physiological responses showcases fasting as a holistic approach to health, addressing not only the physical body but also nurturing cognitive function, hormonal balance, and vital systems such as the gut. In the chapters ahead, we will explore practical aspects of incorporating therapeutic fasting into your lifestyle, ensuring a well-informed and transformative journey toward optimal well-being.

CHAPTER 3: GETTING STARTED WITH THERAPEUTIC FASTING

Embarking on a journey of therapeutic fasting requires thoughtful preparation, a clear understanding of individual goals, and dispelling common misconceptions. In this chapter, we will explore the essential steps to initiate your fasting experience, addressing both the mental and physical aspects of this transformative practice.

1. PREPARING FOR A FAST: MENTAL AND PHYSICAL CONSIDERATIONS:

1.1 Mental Preparation:

Before entering a fasting period, it's crucial to cultivate a positive and informed mindset. Mental preparation involves setting clear intentions, understanding the potential challenges, and adopting a patient and accepting attitude towards the fasting process. Engaging in mindfulness practices, such as meditation or deep breathing exercises, can help foster a sense of calm and focus.

1.2 Physical Preparation:

Physically preparing for a fast involves ensuring your body is adequately nourished leading up to the fasting period. Gradually reducing the intake of processed foods, caffeine, and sugars in the days preceding the fast can help minimize withdrawal symptoms and ease the transition into a fasting state. Staying well-hydrated is equally important, as proper hydration supports the body's detoxification processes.

2. CHOOSING THE RIGHT TYPE OF FAST FOR YOUR GOALS:

2.1 Assessing Personal Goals:

Understanding your health objectives is key to selecting the most suitable fasting approach. Whether your goal is weight management, improved metabolic health, or enhanced mental clarity, aligning the type and duration of your fast with your specific objectives ensures a more tailored and effective experience.

2.2 Exploring Fasting Protocols:

Explore the various fasting protocols, such as intermittent fasting, water fasting, or juice fasting, and assess which aligns best with your preferences and lifestyle. Each protocol offers unique benefits, and selecting the one that resonates with your goals and comfort level enhances the likelihood of a successful and sustainable fasting practice.

3. COMMON MISCONCEPTIONS AND CONCERNS:

3.1 Addressing Nutritional Concerns:

One prevalent misconception is the fear of nutrient deficiencies during fasting. Understanding that well-planned fasts can provide the body with sufficient nutrients and that the focus is on quality over quantity helps alleviate nutritional concerns. Supplements or fortified beverages can also complement fasting periods.

3.2 Overcoming the Fear of Hunger:

The fear of hunger often deters individuals from attempting therapeutic fasting. However, recognizing that hunger is a natural and temporary sensation during fasting, and that the body adapts to this state, can empower individuals to navigate through these moments with ease.

3.3 Dispelling Myths about Energy Levels:

Contrary to the belief that fasting leads to fatigue, many individuals experience increased energy levels and mental clarity during fasting periods. Addressing the myth of reduced energy can instill confidence in those new to the practice.

By meticulously preparing both mentally and physically, selecting an appropriate fasting protocol, and dispelling common misconceptions, you set the stage for a fulfilling and transformative experience. In the subsequent chapters, we will delve into the specifics of different fasting protocols and provide practical guidance on navigating the challenges and maximizing the benefits of therapeutic fasting.

CHAPTER 4: FASTING PROTOCOLS

In the world of therapeutic fasting, various protocols offer individuals flexibility in choosing an approach that aligns with their preferences and health goals. Understanding the nuances of different fasting methods is essential for tailoring your fasting experience to suit your unique needs. In this chapter, we will explore three prominent fasting protocols: Intermittent Fasting, Extended Water Fasting, and other approaches such as Juice Fasting and Partial Fasting.

1. INTERMITTENT FASTING: METHODS AND VARIATIONS:

1.1 16/8 Method:

One of the most popular forms of intermittent fasting, the 16/8 method involves fasting for 16 hours and restricting eating to an 8-hour window. This approach is adaptable to various lifestyles and can be easily incorporated by adjusting the timing of meals.

1.2 5:2 Method:

The 5:2 method involves consuming a regular diet for five days a week and drastically reducing caloric intake (typically around 500-600 calories) on two non-consecutive days. This approach allows for intermittent periods of more substantial caloric restriction.

1.3 Eat-Stop-Eat:

This method involves a complete 24-hour fast once or twice a week. For example, an individual may eat dinner and then abstain from food until the following dinner. The flexibility in choosing fasting days provides ease of integration into different lifestyles.

2. EXTENDED WATER FASTING: GUIDELINES AND SAFETY PRECAUTIONS:

2.1 Understanding Extended Water Fasting:

Extended water fasting typically involves abstaining from all forms of caloric intake and relying solely on water for an extended period. Common durations range from 24 hours to several days, with some individuals opting for longer fasts lasting multiple weeks.

2.2 Guidelines for Extended Water Fasting:

Gradual Preparation: Gradually reduce food intake in the days leading up to an extended water fast.

Adequate Hydration: Ensure proper hydration by drinking ample water throughout the fasting period to support the body's detoxification processes.

Rest and Relaxation: Allow for sufficient rest and avoid strenuous activities during extended water fasting to conserve energy for healing and repair.

2.3 Safety Precautions:

Medical Supervision: Individuals with pre-existing health conditions or those new to extended fasting should seek medical advice and supervision.

Break the Fast Mindfully: Gradually reintroduce food after an extended water fast with easily digestible and nutrient-dense options.

3. OTHER FASTING APPROACHES (E.G., JUICE FASTING, PARTIAL FASTING):

3.1 Juice Fasting:

Juice fasting involves consuming fresh fruit and vegetable juices while abstaining from solid food. This approach provides essential nutrients while still allowing the digestive system to rest. It's crucial to use freshly pressed, high-quality juices for optimal benefits.

3.2 Partial Fasting:

Partial fasting allows for the consumption of a reduced number of calories on specific fasting days. This approach provides more flexibility, making it accessible for individuals who may find complete abstinence challenging. It may involve consuming a limited number of meals or reducing caloric intake on designated days.

As you explore these fasting protocols, it's essential to choose the approach that aligns with your goals, preferences, and overall health. In the following chapters, we will delve into the specific benefits and considerations associated with each fasting method, empowering you to make informed decisions on your therapeutic fasting journey.

CHAPTER 5: LISTENING TO YOUR BODY

In the intricate dance of therapeutic fasting, paying close attention to your body's signals is paramount. The ability to tune into subtle cues ensures a balanced and sustainable fasting experience. In this chapter, we will explore the art of listening to your body during therapeutic fasting, covering essential aspects such as recognizing signs that it's time to break a fast, understanding hunger cues, and adapting fasting protocols to meet individual needs.

1. SIGNS THAT IT'S TIME TO BREAK A FAST:

1.1 Physical Fatigue:
Feeling excessively tired or fatigued can be a sign that your body needs nourishment. If fatigue persists despite adequate rest, it may be an indication to consider breaking your fast.

1.2 Dizziness or Lightheadedness:
Experiencing dizziness or lightheadedness can suggest low blood sugar levels. If these sensations arise, it's essential to prioritize your safety and consider breaking your fast with a nutritious meal.

1.3 Persistent Headaches:

Fasting-induced headaches may occur, but if they persist and become severe, it's crucial to interpret them as a signal from your body. Breaking the fast and replenishing essential nutrients may alleviate this symptom.

1.4 Gastrointestinal Discomfort:

Persistent stomach pains or discomfort can indicate that your digestive system requires attention. Breaking the fast with easily digestible foods can provide relief and prevent further discomfort.

2. UNDERSTANDING HUNGER CUES DURING FASTING:

2.1 Distinguishing Between True Hunger and Cravings:

True hunger typically manifests gradually and may be accompanied by physical sensations like stomach rumbling. Distinguishing between true hunger and cravings is essential for making informed decisions about when to break a fast.

2.2 Emotional Hunger vs. Physical Hunger:

Understanding the emotional aspects of hunger is crucial during fasting. Emotional hunger may stem from stress, boredom, or other non-physical factors. Learning to differentiate between emotional and physical hunger can guide your response to hunger cues.

2.3 Cognitive Clarity vs. Cognitive Fog:

Consider the mental aspect of hunger cues. While some individuals experience heightened cognitive clarity during fasting, others may encounter cognitive fog. Recognizing shifts in mental acuity can guide your decision-making regarding the continuation or conclusion of a fast.

3. ADJUSTING FASTING PROTOCOLS

BASED ON INDIVIDUAL NEEDS:

3.1 Assessing Energy Levels:

Regularly assess your energy levels throughout the fasting period. If you notice a persistent decline in energy, it may be an indicator to modify your fasting approach, either by adjusting the duration or choosing a different fasting protocol.

3.2 Personalizing Fasting Duration:

Fasting is not one-size-fits-all. Personalizing your fasting duration based on your body's response and your individual goals is a key component of a successful and sustainable fasting practice.

3.3 Navigating Hormonal Changes:

Individual responses to fasting can vary, particularly in terms of hormonal changes. Pay attention to how your body reacts to fasting, especially concerning hormonal balance, and consider adjustments as needed.

Listening to your body is an ongoing and dynamic process during therapeutic fasting. By recognizing the signs that indicate the need to break a fast, understanding the nuances of hunger cues, and adapting fasting protocols based on individual needs, you empower yourself to cultivate a mindful and harmonious relationship with the transformative practice of therapeutic fasting. In the subsequent chapters, we will delve deeper into the intricacies of fasting, offering practical insights to guide your journey toward optimal well-being.

CHAPTER 6: COMBINING THERAPEUTIC FASTING WITH OTHER LIFESTYLE PRACTICES

As you embrace the transformative power of therapeutic fasting, synergizing this practice with other elements of a healthy lifestyle becomes instrumental in maximizing its benefits. In this chapter, we will explore the integration of fasting with a balanced diet, the importance of incorporating exercise and stress management, and how sleep plays a crucial role in the fasting process.

1. INTEGRATING FASTING WITH A BALANCED DIET:

1.1 Understanding Nutrient-Dense Foods:

Complementing your fasting periods with a balanced and nutrient-dense diet is essential for overall well-being. When breaking a fast, prioritize whole foods rich in vitamins, minerals, and essential nutrients. This approach not only supports your body's nutritional needs but also enhances the positive outcomes of fasting.

1.2 Mindful Eating Practices:

Practicing mindfulness during meals contributes to a more conscious and enjoyable eating experience. Chew your food thoroughly, savor each bite, and listen to your body's satiety cues.

This mindful approach fosters a healthier relationship with food and complements the holistic benefits of therapeutic fasting.

1.3 Hydration and Electrolyte Balance:

Maintaining proper hydration is crucial, especially during fasting periods. Water, herbal teas, and broths can support hydration, while electrolytes such as sodium, potassium, and magnesium help balance essential minerals. Ensuring adequate hydration and electrolyte balance supports your body's functions and mitigates potential side effects of fasting.

2. INCORPORATING EXERCISE AND STRESS MANAGEMENT:

2.1 Moderate Exercise during Fasting:

Engaging in moderate physical activity during fasting periods can enhance the metabolic effects of fasting. Activities like walking, yoga, or light aerobic exercises contribute to overall well-being without placing excessive strain on the body.

2.2 Stress Management Strategies:

Stress management is a crucial component of a holistic approach to health. Incorporate stress-reducing practices such as meditation, deep breathing exercises, or mindfulness activities into your routine. These practices complement therapeutic fasting by promoting a balanced and harmonious internal environment.

2.3 Balancing Rest and Movement:

Find the equilibrium between rest and movement. While incorporating physical activity is beneficial, ensuring adequate rest and recovery is equally important. Balancing rest and movement supports your body's ability to adapt to the fasting process and fosters a sustainable and balanced lifestyle.

3. SLEEP AND ITS ROLE IN THE FASTING PROCESS:

3.1 Prioritizing Quality Sleep:

Quality sleep is foundational to overall well-being, and its importance is magnified during therapeutic fasting. Aim for a consistent sleep schedule, create a calming bedtime routine, and ensure a comfortable sleep environment to optimize the restorative benefits of sleep.

3.2 Circadian Rhythms and Fasting:

Aligning fasting periods with natural circadian rhythms can enhance the efficacy of therapeutic fasting. Consider timing your fasting windows to coincide with your body's natural fasting and feeding cycles for a more seamless integration into your daily routine.

3.3 The Synergy of Sleep and Fasting:

Sleep and fasting share a symbiotic relationship. Quality sleep supports hormonal balance, cognitive function, and overall metabolic health, reinforcing the positive effects of therapeutic fasting. Conversely, a well-implemented fasting practice can contribute to improved sleep quality over time.

By integrating therapeutic fasting with a balanced diet, incorporating mindful eating practices, embracing moderate exercise and stress management, and prioritizing quality sleep, you create a comprehensive and synergistic approach to health. In the subsequent chapters, we will delve deeper into practical strategies and tips to support your journey, ensuring a harmonious and sustainable incorporation of therapeutic fasting into your lifestyle.

CHAPTER 7: COMMON CHALLENGES AND SOLUTIONS

As you embark on the journey of therapeutic fasting, it's essential to anticipate and navigate common challenges that may arise. This chapter will delve into practical solutions for dealing with potential side effects, addressing social and cultural aspects of fasting, and troubleshooting difficulties and setbacks along the way.

1. DEALING WITH POTENTIAL SIDE EFFECTS:

1.1 Understanding Common Side Effects:

Therapeutic fasting can sometimes bring about side effects as your body adjusts to the changes. Common side effects may include headaches, fatigue, dizziness, or digestive discomfort. Recognizing these symptoms allows for proactive management.

1.2 Adequate Hydration:

Many side effects can be mitigated by maintaining proper hydration. Ensure you drink enough water, herbal teas, and electrolyte-rich fluids to support your body during fasting periods. Staying hydrated aids in reducing potential headaches, dizziness, and fatigue.

1.3 Gradual Adaptation:

If you experience persistent side effects, consider a gradual adaptation approach. Start with shorter fasting durations and progressively extend them as your body acclimates to the practice. This allows for a gentler introduction to therapeutic fasting.

2. ADDRESSING SOCIAL AND CULTURAL ASPECTS OF FASTING:

2.1 Communication and Education:

Open communication with friends, family, and colleagues is crucial. Educate them about the purpose and benefits of therapeutic fasting to foster understanding and support. Clearly communicate your goals and the importance of maintaining a positive and non-judgmental environment.

2.2 Participating Mindfully in Social Events:

Social gatherings often revolve around shared meals. When participating in such events, plan ahead and make informed choices. Opt for nutrient-dense foods, or if needed, consider breaking your fast temporarily to align with the social context. Striking a balance allows you to enjoy social occasions without compromising your fasting goals.

2.3 Cultivating a Support System:

Surround yourself with a supportive network. Share your fasting journey with like-minded individuals or seek communities that embrace similar practices. Having a support system provides encouragement, advice, and a sense of camaraderie.

3. TROUBLESHOOTING DIFFICULTIES AND SETBACKS:

3.1 Reassessing Fasting Protocols:

If you encounter difficulties, reassess your fasting protocols. Consider adjusting the duration, type of fast, or incorporating refeeding days to provide your body with additional nutrients. Tailoring your approach based on your experiences ensures a more adaptable and sustainable fasting practice.

3.2 Mindful Reflection:

When setbacks occur, engage in mindful reflection rather than self-criticism. Assess the factors contributing to the setback and use it as an opportunity for learning and growth. Cultivating a positive mindset supports resilience in overcoming challenges.

3.3 Seeking Professional Guidance:

If difficulties persist or if you have underlying health concerns, seek guidance from healthcare professionals or nutritionists experienced in therapeutic fasting. Professional advice ensures a personalized approach that aligns with your health goals and addresses specific challenges you may be facing.

Navigating common challenges is an integral part of the therapeutic fasting journey. By proactively addressing potential side effects, fostering understanding in social and cultural contexts, and troubleshooting difficulties with adaptability and support, you empower yourself to overcome obstacles and continue on the path toward optimal well-being. In the following chapters, we will delve into advanced strategies and long-term considerations, further enhancing your mastery of therapeutic fasting.

CHAPTER 8: SUCCESS STORIES

In the realm of therapeutic fasting, success stories abound, each representing a unique journey towards improved health and well-being. In this chapter, we will explore real-life examples of individuals who have experienced transformative benefits through therapeutic fasting, showcasing the diverse experiences and outcomes that underscore the potential of this practice.

1. REAL-LIFE EXAMPLES OF INDIVIDUALS WHO HAVE BENEFITED FROM THERAPEUTIC FASTING:

1.1 Weight Management Triumphs:

Meet Sarah, a dedicated mother who struggled with weight management for years. Through the implementation of intermittent fasting, Sarah discovered a sustainable approach that not only helped her shed excess pounds but also provided a newfound sense of control over her eating habits. Her success story highlights the adaptability of therapeutic fasting in addressing weight-related challenges.

1.2 Improved Metabolic Health:

John, a middle-aged professional, experienced remarkable improvements in his metabolic health through extended water fasting. Despite initial skepticism, John's commitment to the practice led to enhanced insulin sensitivity, normalized blood sugar levels, and a significant reduction in markers of inflammation. His journey exemplifies the power of therapeutic fasting in promoting metabolic well-being.

1.3 Cognitive Clarity and Mental Resilience:

Emma, a college student facing the pressures of academic life, found solace in therapeutic fasting. Adopting intermittent fasting, Emma noticed heightened cognitive clarity, improved focus, and enhanced mental resilience. Her success story illustrates the cognitive benefits that can accompany a well-balanced fasting practice.

2. DIVERSE EXPERIENCES AND OUTCOMES:

2.1 Personalized Approaches to Fasting:

Explore the story of Alex, who embraced a personalized approach to fasting based on his individual needs and preferences. By experimenting with different fasting protocols, Alex discovered a regimen that seamlessly integrated into his lifestyle, resulting in sustained benefits without sacrificing enjoyment.

2.2 Overcoming Chronic Health Issues:

Jasmine, dealing with chronic health issues, sought relief through therapeutic fasting. Her journey involved a combination of intermittent fasting and targeted dietary changes. Over time, Jasmine experienced a reduction in symptoms, improved energy levels, and an overall sense of well-being, showcasing the potential of fasting in addressing various health challenges.

2.3 Enhanced Athletic Performance:

Discover Mark's success story, an athlete who leveraged therapeutic fasting to enhance his physical performance. Mark's experience demonstrates how strategic fasting protocols can optimize energy utilization, improve endurance, and support overall athletic goals.

These real-life success stories exemplify the diverse ways in which individuals have harnessed the benefits of therapeutic fasting to transform their lives. As you navigate your own journey, consider these narratives as sources of inspiration and insight. Remember that each person's experience is unique, and the key lies in discovering the fasting approach that aligns with your goals, preferences, and individual needs.

CHAPTER 10: FREQUENTLY ASKED QUESTIONS (FAQS)

As you delve into the world of therapeutic fasting, it's natural to have questions and concerns. This chapter aims to address common queries and alleviate any uncertainties you may have about this transformative practice.

1. How do I choose the right fasting method for me?

Choosing the right fasting method depends on your health goals, lifestyle, and individual preferences. Consider factors such as your current health status, the desired outcome of fasting, and how well a particular fasting protocol aligns with your daily routine. Experimenting with different approaches and monitoring how your body responds will help you find the method that suits you best.

2. Is therapeutic fasting safe for everyone?

While therapeutic fasting can be beneficial for many individuals, it may not be suitable for everyone. Individuals with certain medical conditions, pregnant or breastfeeding women, and those with a history of eating disorders should consult with a healthcare professional before embarking on a fasting journey. Seeking professional guidance ensures that the practice aligns with your unique health circumstances.

3. How do I manage hunger during fasting?

Managing hunger during fasting involves understanding the difference between true hunger and cravings. Staying well-hydrated, engaging in activities to distract the mind, and consuming beverages like herbal teas can help curb hunger sensations. Additionally, gradual adaptation and choosing a fasting method that aligns with your lifestyle can make it easier to manage hunger over time.

4. Can I exercise while fasting?

Yes, you can exercise during fasting periods. In fact, incorporating moderate exercise can enhance the benefits of therapeutic fasting. Activities such as walking, yoga, or light aerobic exercises are generally well-tolerated during fasting. However, it's essential to listen to your body and adjust the intensity of your workouts based on how you feel.

5. What should I eat when breaking a fast?

When breaking a fast, focus on nutrient-dense foods to provide your body with essential vitamins and minerals. Opt for whole foods, including fruits, vegetables, lean proteins, and healthy fats. Avoid consuming large or heavy meals immediately after fasting, and instead, start with smaller, easily digestible portions to allow your digestive system to adjust gradually.

6. Can therapeutic fasting help with weight loss?

Yes, therapeutic fasting can be an effective tool for weight loss. By creating a caloric deficit during fasting periods, the body taps into stored fat for energy, leading to weight loss over time. Combining fasting with a balanced diet and regular physical activity enhances the potential for sustainable weight management.

7. How long should I fast for optimal benefits?

The optimal duration of fasting varies among individuals and depends on personal goals. Intermittent fasting methods, such as the 16/8 or 5:2 approaches, involve shorter durations and may be more sustainable for some. Extended water fasts lasting 24 hours to several days offer deeper metabolic benefits but require careful consideration and supervision. It's essential to find a duration that aligns with your goals and feels manageable for you.

8. Can therapeutic fasting be done long-term?

The feasibility of long-term therapeutic fasting depends on individual factors, including overall health, goals, and lifestyle. While intermittent fasting can often be incorporated into a long-term lifestyle, extended water fasts may be more suitable as occasional practices. Consistency, adaptation, and regular health check-ups are key factors in determining the sustainability of therapeutic fasting over the long term.

9. What if I experience adverse effects during fasting?

If you experience adverse effects, such as persistent dizziness, severe fatigue, or gastrointestinal discomfort, it's crucial to listen to your body and consider breaking your fast. Gradual adaptation, proper hydration, and seeking professional advice can help address potential adverse effects. If symptoms persist or worsen, consult with a healthcare professional to ensure a safe and tailored approach to therapeutic fasting.

10. Can therapeutic fasting help with specific health conditions?

Therapeutic fasting has shown potential benefits for various health conditions, including metabolic disorders, inflammation-related issues, and certain chronic diseases. However, the impact may vary among individuals, and it's important to consult with a healthcare professional before using therapeutic fasting as a primary intervention for specific health conditions. Professional guidance ensures that fasting aligns with your overall health management plan.

Remember, the information provided in this eBook is a guide, and individual responses to therapeutic fasting may differ. It's advisable to consult with healthcare professionals or nutritionists, especially if you have pre-existing health conditions or concerns about integrating fasting into your lifestyle. With careful consideration and personalized adjustments, therapeutic fasting can be a valuable tool on your journey toward optimal well-being.

CHAPTER 10: RESOURCES AND FURTHER READING

For readers eager to delve deeper into the world of therapeutic fasting, a wealth of resources awaits. This chapter compiles a curated list of additional references, books, and websites that can serve as valuable companions on your journey toward understanding, implementing, and mastering the art of therapeutic fasting.

1. BOOKS ON THERAPEUTIC FASTING:

"The Complete Guide to Fasting: Heal Your Body Through Intermittent, Alternate-Day, and Extended Fasting" by Dr. Jason Fung and Jimmy Moore: A comprehensive guide that explores various fasting methods, their benefits, and practical tips for implementation.

"The Obesity Code: Unlocking the Secrets of Weight Loss" by Dr. Jason Fung: Dr. Fung delves into the underlying causes of obesity and presents a paradigm-shifting perspective on weight management, incorporating principles of intermittent fasting.

"The Longevity Diet: Discover the New Science Behind Stem Cell Activation and Regeneration to Slow Aging, Fight Disease, and Optimize Weight" by Dr. Valter Longo: Dr. Longo explores the connection between fasting, cellular regeneration, and longevity, providing insights into the science behind therapeutic fasting.

2. WEBSITES AND ONLINE RESOURCES:

Dr. Jason Fung's Blog: Dr. Fung's blog offers in-depth articles, research summaries, and practical advice on therapeutic fasting, intermittent fasting, and metabolic health.

The Fasting Method: An online platform co-founded by Dr. Jason Fung and Megan Ramos, providing resources, courses, and community support for individuals interested in therapeutic fasting.

The IDM Program: The Institute for Diabetes and Metabolic Health, founded by Dr. Jason Fung, offers educational materials, webinars, and resources related to therapeutic fasting and metabolic health.

3. SCIENTIFIC JOURNALS AND ARTICLES:

"Intermittent Fasting: Surprising Update" by Dr. Michael Mosley: Dr. Mosley explores the latest findings on intermittent fasting and its potential health benefits in this insightful article.

"Effects of Intermittent Fasting on Health, Aging, and Disease" - New England Journal of Medicine: A comprehensive review article that examines the effects of intermittent fasting on various health aspects, published in the New England Journal of Medicine.

4. PODCASTS AND INTERVIEWS:

The Fasting Talk Podcast: Hosted by Jimmy Moore, this podcast features insightful discussions with experts in the field of therapeutic fasting, covering a wide range of topics.

The Drive with Dr. Peter Attia: Dr. Peter Attia's podcast delves into the realms of longevity, metabolic health, and fasting through engaging interviews with leading experts.

5. ONLINE COMMUNITIES:

r/fasting (Reddit): An active online community where individuals share their experiences, ask questions, and provide support related to various fasting methods.

Facebook Groups: Numerous Facebook groups centered around therapeutic fasting and intermittent fasting provide spaces for sharing stories, insights, and advice.

As you explore these resources, remember that knowledge is a dynamic and evolving journey. Continuously seek reliable information, stay open to new perspectives, and tailor your approach to suit your individual needs. The world of therapeutic fasting is rich with insights and discoveries waiting to be explored.

CONCLUSION

As you reach the end of this journey through the pages of our exploration into therapeutic fasting, take a moment to reflect on the key concepts that have unfolded. From understanding the science behind fasting to navigating its diverse protocols, addressing common concerns, and delving into real-life success stories, you've acquired a foundation that empowers you on your path to optimal well-being.

RECAP OF KEY CONCEPTS:

Understanding Therapeutic Fasting: You've gained insights into the science behind therapeutic fasting, recognizing its potential to promote metabolic health, weight management, and cognitive well-being.

Fasting Protocols: Explore a spectrum of fasting protocols, from intermittent fasting to extended water fasting and other variations, allowing you to tailor your approach based on personal preferences and goals.

Listening to Your Body: The art of tuning into your body's signals during fasting emerged as a pivotal theme. Recognizing signs to break a fast, understanding hunger cues, and adjusting protocols based on individual needs are crucial skills.

Combining Fasting with Lifestyle Practices: Integrating fasting with a balanced diet, incorporating exercise, managing stress, and prioritizing quality sleep emerged as holistic strategies for maximizing the benefits of therapeutic fasting.

Common Challenges and Solutions: Acknowledging potential side effects, addressing social and cultural aspects, and troubleshooting setbacks underscored the importance of adaptability and resilience in your fasting journey.

Success Stories: Real-life examples showcased the transformative potential of therapeutic fasting, illustrating diverse experiences and outcomes that inspire and inform your own unique path.

Frequently Asked Questions: Addressing common concerns provided clarity and guidance, offering practical solutions to questions that may arise on your fasting journey.

ENCOURAGEMENT AND MOTIVATION FOR YOUR FASTING JOURNEY:

Embarking on a journey of therapeutic fasting is a personal and transformative experience. As you venture forward, let encouragement be your companion. Embrace the knowledge you've gained, but also remember that this is a journey of self-discovery, adaptation, and growth.

You Are Not Alone: Whether you are just starting or have been practicing therapeutic fasting for a while, remember that you are not alone on this journey. Communities, both online and offline, offer support, shared experiences, and valuable insights. Connect with like-minded individuals who can inspire and encourage you along the way.

Embrace Progress, Not Perfection: Your fasting journey

is a dynamic process. Embrace progress over perfection, acknowledging that each step forward is a testament to your commitment to well-being. Be patient with yourself, celebrate small victories, and learn from challenges.

Listen to Your Body: Your body is a guide on this journey. Listen to its cues, be attuned to its signals, and make adjustments as needed. The beauty of therapeutic fasting lies in its adaptability—tailor your approach based on how your body responds, ensuring a sustainable and enjoyable experience.

Celebrate Your Unique Path: Each individual's journey with therapeutic fasting is inherently unique. Celebrate the diversity of experiences and outcomes, recognizing that your path may differ from others. What matters most is the positive impact it has on your overall health and well-being.

As you take these closing words with you, may they serve as a source of inspiration and empowerment. Your journey with therapeutic fasting is a testament to your commitment to a healthier and more balanced life. Wishing you resilience, curiosity, and fulfillment on your continued path of discovery and well-being.

ABOUT THE AUTHOR

Promise Adebayo

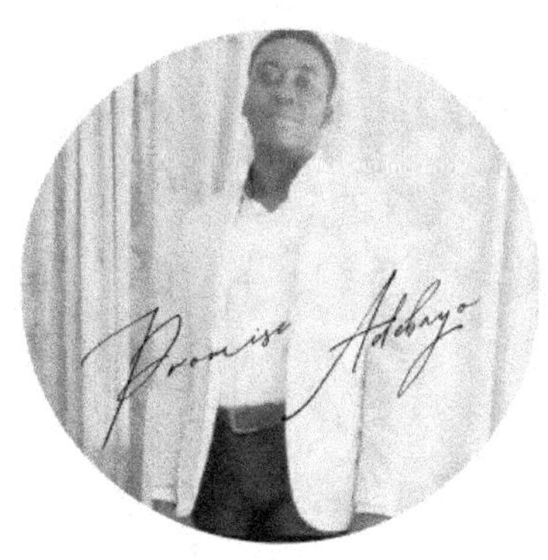

PROMISE ADEBAYO], the author of "Therapeutic Fasting: Unlocking the Healing Powers of Abstinence," is a passionate advocate for holistic well-being and an avid researcher in the field of health and nutrition. With a background in Health Topics, PROMISE brings a unique blend of scientific knowledge and practical insights to guide readers on their journey towards optimal health.

Driven by a genuine commitment to share transformative practices, PROMISE has dedicated years to studying and understanding the profound benefits of therapeutic fasting. This Book is a culmination of that journey, aiming to demystify the intricacies of fasting and empower readers to harness its healing powers in a mindful and sustainable way.

As you delve into the pages of "Therapeutic Fasting," consider PROMISE as your knowledgeable guide, accompanying you on a journey toward a healthier, more vibrant life. May the insights shared in this eBook be a valuable resource on your path to discovering the transformative potential of therapeutic fasting.